Little

Book

Of

Fitness

Quotes

Thank you to all of the amazing coaches, teammates, mentors, and role models that I have come across in my journey thus far. You have all inspired me to push harder, dig deeper, and keep on working when the going gets tough in both sports and in life.

Fitness and health are topics that most of us can relate to. I was never one of those athletes that seemed to have some innate talent given to them at birth; I have had to work extremely hard for everything I achieved. I am here to tell you: keep on working hard every day and never give up on your dreams... anything is possible through persistence.

This book contains a list of 365+ Fitness quotes from all over the world to help motivate, inspire, and push you to get into the best shape you can possibly be.

These quotes come from a wide range of top Fitness celebrities, authors, personal trainers, body builders, and motivational speakers. I have left out all company names, brands, and logos.

Read one every morning to start your day off on the right foot in a positive mindset before the world has a chance to beat you down and play with your emotions.

The most powerful way to improve your Fitness performance is to first change your way of thinking, and this book will help you with that. Read a quote every day, absorbing knowledge from the best people in the Fitness world!

"An investment in knowledge pays the best interest."
—Benjamin Franklin

1. There is a difference between interest and commitment. When you are interested in doing something, you only do it when it's convenient. When you are committed to something, you accept no excuses, only results.
   —Ken Blanchard

2. Your legs are not giving out... your head is giving up.
   —Unknown

3. Lack of activity destroys the good condition of every human being, while movement and methodical physical exercise save it and preserve it. —Plato

4. Work hard in silence, let success make the noise. —Frank Ocean

5. Discipline is choosing between what you want now and what you want most. —Abraham Lincoln

6. If you have a body, you are an athlete. —Bill Bowerman

7. To keep the body in good health is a duty, for otherwise we shall not be able to trim the lamp of wisdom, and keep our mind strong and clear. Water surrounds the lotus flower, but does not wet its petals. —Buddha

8. Set goals and then kick them in the face! —Unknown

9. I just woke up one day and decided I didn't want to feel like that anymore, or ever again. So I changed... just like that. —Unknown

10. Someone much busier than you is working out right now. —Unknown

11. Crawling, falling, puking, crying, blood, and pain are all acceptable... quitting is not! —Unknown

12. Things work out best for those who make the best of how things work out. —John Wooden

13. I feel an endless need to learn, to improve, to evolve - not only to please the coach and the fans - but also to feel satisfied with myself. –Christiano Ronaldo

14. Too many people confine their exercise to jumping to conclusions, running up bills, stretching the truth, bending over backward, lying down on the job, sidestepping responsibility and pushing their luck. –Unknown

15. If you were able to believe in Santa Claus for like 8 years, you can believe in yourself for 5 minutes. –Unknown

16. My heart says chocolate and wine, but my pants say for the love of god have a salad and go to the gym.
    —Unknown

17. Don't compare your beginning to someone else's middle or end. —Jon Acuff

18. The only thing standing between you and your goal is the bullshit story you keep telling yourself as to why you can't achieve it.
    —Grant Cardone

19. In training, you listen to your body. In competition, you tell your body to shut up. —Rich Froning Jr.

20. Ninety-nine percent of the failures come from people who have the habit of making excuses.
—George Washington

21. There are no secrets to success. It is the result of preparation, hard work, and learning from failure.
—Colin Powell

22. Work out, eat well, and be patient. Your body will reward you. —Unknown

23. Giving up on your goal because of one setback is like slashing your other three tires because you got one flat. —Unknown

24. Leave all the afternoon for exercise and recreation, which are as necessary as reading. I should rather say more necessary because health is worth more than learning. —Thomas Jefferson

25. Exercise to be fit, not skinny. Eat to nourish your body and always ignore the haters, doubters, and unhealthy examples that were once feeding you. You are worth more than you realize. —Unknown

26. If you focus on results, you will never change. If you focus on change, you will get results. —Jack Dixon

27. Take time to deliberate, but when the time for action has arrived, stop thinking and go in.
—Napolean Bonaparte

28. Everyone must choose one of two pains: the pain of discipline or the pain of regret. -Jim Rohn

29. If you always put limits on everything you do, physical or anything else, it will spread into your work and into your life. There are no limits. There are only plateaus; and you must not stay there, you must go beyond them. -Bruce Lee

30. Just stick with it. What seems hard now will one day be your warm up. —Unknown

31. Some people want it to happen, some wish it would happen, others make it happen. —Michael Jordan

32. Wake up every morning with determination, go to bed with satisfaction! —George Lorimer

33. My doctor recently told me that jogging could add years to my life. I think he was right. I feel ten years older already. —Milton Berle

34. We must appreciate and never underestimate our own inner power.
—Noah Galloway

35. Water, air, and cleanliness are the chief articles in my pharmacopoeia. —Napoleon

36. It's not who you think you are that holds you back; it's who you think you're not.
—Unknown

37. Second by second, you lose the opportunity to become the person you want to be. When are you going to stop making excuses and take charge of your life?
—Greg Pitt

38. There's no secret formula. I lift heavy, work hard, and aim to be the best.
    —Ronnie Coleman

39. Time and health are two precious assets that we don't recognize and appreciate until they have been depleted. —Denis Waitley

40. If you wait for perfect conditions, you will never get anything done.
    —Unknown

41. The struggle you are in today is developing the strength you need for tomorrow. —Robert Tew

42. The deviation of man from the state in which he was originally placed by nature seems to have proved to him a prolific source of diseases.
   —Edward Jenner

43. Many so-called spiritual people, they overeat, drink too much, they smoke and don't exercise. But they do go to church every week and pray *"Please help my arthritis. Please help me bring up my strength, make me young again"*.
   —Jack LaLanne

44. If your dog is fat, you're not getting enough exercise.
   —Unknown

45. A 30 minute workout is just two percent of your day. No excuses! —Unknown

46. I tried every diet in the book. I tried some that weren't in the book. I tried eating the book. It tasted better than most of the diets. —Dolly Parton

47. One pound of fat is 3,500 calories. If you want to lose one pound a week, just burn 500 more calories a day than you eat. Fitness is a science, not magic. —Unknown

48. Of all the hazards, fear is the worst. —Sam Snead

49. A man too busy to take care of his health is like a mechanic too busy to take care of his tools.
    —Spanish Proverb

50. My own prescription for health is less paperwork and more running barefoot through the grass.
    —Leslie Grimutter

51. A number on a scale does not dictate your health or your worth. —Unknown

52. An hour of basketball feels like 15 minutes. An hour on the treadmill feels like a weekend at traffic school.
    —David Walters

53. The greatest wealth is health. —Virgil

54. To love yourself is to understand you don't need to be perfect to be good. —Unknown

55. You can't depend on your eyes when your imagination is out of focus. —Mark Twain

56. Never give up on a dream just because of the time it will take to accomplish it. The time will pass anyway. —Earl Nightingale

57. Fitness is like a marriage. You can't cheat on it and expect it to work. —Unknown

58. You have a choice. You can throw in the towel or you can use it to wipe the sweat off your face. —Unknown

59. Walking: the most ancient exercise and still the best modern exercise.
    —Carrie Latet

60. Mainstream medicine would be way different if they focused on prevention even half as much as they focused on intervention. —Unknown

61. When you stop chasing the wrong things, you give the right things a chance to catch you. —Lolly Daskal

62. Set some goals, then demolish them. Then set new goals, and destroy those. —Miko

63. Nobody is perfect, so get over the fear of being or doing everything perfectly. Besides, perfect is boring. —Jillian Michaels

64. Anything is possible if you've got enough nerve. —J.K. Rowling

65. You won't always love the workout, but you'll always love the results. —Unknown

66. When you feel like quitting, think about why you started in the first place. —Unknown

67. If doubt is challenging you and you do not act, doubts will grow. Challenge the doubts with action and you will grow. Doubt and action are incompatible.
    —John Kanary

68. Most of our obstacles would melt away if, instead of cowering before them, we would make up our minds to walk boldly through them.
    —Orison Swett Marden

69. Strength doesn't come from what you can do. It comes from overcoming the things you once thought you couldn't. —Rikki Rogers

70. When you get right down to the root of the meaning of the word *succeed*, you find that it simply means to follow through.
    −F.W. Nichol

71. Do not stop until that little voice in your head says *"I'm proud of you"*. −Unknown

72. Nothing is impossible, the word itself says *I'm possible*. −Audrey Hepburn

73. I'm not training for a 5k. I'm not preparing for a competition. I'm not trying to set a new record. I'm not trying to impress you. I'm saving my life. −Unknown

74. If something stands between you and your success, move it. Never be denied.
    —Dwayne Johnson

75. I'm not losing weight, I'm getting rid of it... I have no intention of finding it again.
    —Unknown

76. A bad attitude is worse than a bad swing.
    —Payne Stewart

77. Remember this: your body is your slave; it works for you.
    —Jack LaLanne

78. If we wait until we are ready, we will be waiting for the rest of our lives.
    —Lemony Snicket

79. Take up one idea. Make that one idea your life – think of it, dream of it, live on that idea. Let the brain, muscles, nerves, every part of your body, be full of that idea, and just leave every other idea alone. This is the way to success.
    —Swami Vivekananda

80. Your health account, your bank account, they're the same thing. The more you put in, the more you can take out. Exercise is king and nutrition is queen. Together you have a kingdom. —Jack LaLanne

81. Don't think. Just put your shoes on and go for a run. –Unknown

82. There are two primary choices in life: to accept conditions as they exist, or accept the responsibility for changing them. –Dr. Denis Waitley

83. If your spine is inflexibly stiff at 30, you are old. If it is completely flexible at 60, you are young. –Joseph H. Pilates

84. The successful warrior is the average man, with laser-like focus. –Bruce Lee

85. You can do anything for one minute. If you can do it for one, there is a good chance you can do it for two. If you can do it for two, there is a good chance you can do it for three. —Unknown

86. Fitness isn't a seasonal hobby. Fitness is a lifestyle. —Unknown

87. It's never too late... never too late to start over, never too late to be happy. —Jane Fonda

88. Don't say *"I can't"*. Say *"I presently struggle with"*. —Tony Horton

89. Most people give up right before the big break comes – don't let that person be you. –Michael Boyle

90. Stop conforming to the cancer of *can't*. –Unknown

91. To insure good health: eat lightly, breathe deeply, live moderately, cultivate cheerfulness, and maintain an interest in life. –William Londen

92. It's not about having time. It's about making time. People will always find time for what they think is important. –Jeremy Bhimji

93. Nobody cares about your excuses. Nobody pities you for procrastinating. Nobody is going to cuddle you because you are lazy. It's your ass... you move it!
—Unknown

94. Health is a state of complete physical, mental and social well-being, and not merely the absence of disease or infirmity.
—World Health Organization

95. People often say that motivation doesn't last. Well, neither does bathing... that's why we recommend it daily.
—Zig Ziglar

96. I go to the gym because I think my great personality could use a bang'n body.
    –Unknown

97. Enough sleep is just as important for good health as nutrition and exercise.
    –Unknown

98. The only bad workout is the one you didn't do.
    –Unknown

99. Every living cell in your body is made from the food you eat. If you consistently eat junk food then you'll have a junk body. –Jeanette Jenkins

100. Small daily improvements
     are the key to staggering
     long-term results.
     —Unknown

101. Motivation is what gets
     you started. Habit is what
     keeps you going.
     —Jim Ryan

102. A healthy body is a
     platform for a flourishing
     and healthy mind.
     —Pawan Mishra

103. It's easier to wake up early
     in the morning and work
     out, than it is to look in
     the mirror each day and
     not like what you see.
     —Unknown

104. Whether it's ten or one, you will NEVER regret lacing up those running shoes and going outside. —Unknown

105. It's the start that stops most people... don't be most people. —Unknown

106. The journey of a thousand miles begins with a single step. —Lao Tzu

107. No masterpiece was ever created by a lazy artist. —Unknown

108. Don't judge each day by the harvest you reap, but by the seeds you plant. —Robert Louis Stevenson

109. To succeed you must first improve, to improve you must first practice, to practice you must first learn, to learn you must first fail. —Wesley Woo

110. I exercise because somehow completely exhausting myself is the most relaxing part of my day. —Unknown

111. Decide what you want, decide what you are willing to exchange for it. Establish your priorities and go to work. —H.L. Hunt

112. A goal is not always meant to be reached; it often serves simply as something to aim at. —Bruce Lee

113. The body only profits a little from exercising, but the spirit profits a lot. —Billy Blanks

114. As for butter versus margarine, I trust cows more than chemists. —Joan Gussow

115. *Obsessed* is a word the lazy use to describe the dedicated. —Unknown

116. Whether you think you can or think you can't, you are right. —Unknown

117. You can't cross a sea merely by standing and staring at the water.
    —Rabindranath Tagore

118. You must have long-range goals to keep you from being frustrated by short-range failures.
    —Charles C. Noble

119. I already know what giving up feels like. I want to see what happens if I don't.
    —Neila Ray

120. I think you might dispense with half your doctors if you would only consult Dr. Sun more.
    —Henry Ward Beecher

121. Get comfortable with being uncomfortable.
   —Jillian Michaels

122. You shall gain, but you shall pay with sweat, blood, and vomit.
   —Pavel Tsatsouline

123. You didn't come this far only to come this far.
   —Unknown

124. The thing about reaching your goal is that it's 100% possible. It's completely in your control. The only thing stopping you from getting there is you. So get out of the way.
   —Unknown

125. Go as long as you can, and then take another step.
—Unknown

126. The best of all medicines is resting and fasting.
—Benjamin Franklin

127. There are far better things ahead than any we leave behind. —C.S. Lewis

128. Just because you're not sick does not mean you're healthy. —Unknown

129. We run to undo the damage we have done to our body and spirit. We run to find some part of ourselves yet undiscovered.
—John Bingham

130. The only time you should ever look back is to see how far you have come.
—Unknown

131. Today, more than 95% of all chronic disease is caused by food choice, toxic food ingredients, nutritional deficiencies and lack of physical exercise.
—Mike Adams

132. When you are trying to motivate yourself, appreciate the fact that you are even thinking about making a change. And as you move forward, allow yourself to be good enough. —Alice Domar

133. Your struggles develop your strengths. When you go through hardships and decide not to surrender, that is strength.
    —Arnold Schwarzenegger

134. A man can be as great as he wants to be. If you believe in yourself and have the courage, the determination, the dedication, the competitive drive and if you are willing to sacrifice the little things in life and pay the price for the things that are worthwhile, it can be done.
    —Vince Lombardi

135. Wake up every single morning and tell yourself "I can do this"! —Unknown

136. You don't notice it, but every workout is one step closer to your goals. —Unknown

137. Change comes from self-love, not self-loathing. —Lauren Fleshman

138. If you don't do what's best for your body, you're the one who comes up on the short end. —Julius Erving

139. The elevator to success is out of order. You'll have to use the stairs... one at a time. —Joe Girard

140. How different our lives are when we really know what is deeply important to us, and keeping that picture in mind, we manage ourselves each day to be and to do what really matters most.
    —Stephen Covey

141. The older you get, the tougher it is to lose weight because by then, your body and your fat are really good friends.
    —Anonymous

142. Fit is not a destination. It's a way of life. —Unknown

143. If you ain't pissed off for greatness, that just means you're okay with being mediocre. —Ray Lewis

144. Do what you have to do until you can do what you want to do! —Oprah

145. The strongest oak tree of the forest is not the one that is protected from the storm and hidden from the sun. It's the one that stands in the open where it is compelled to struggle for its existence against the winds and rains and the scorching sun.
—Napoleon Hill

146. Most of us think we don't have enough time to exercise. What a distorted paradigm! We don't have time *not* to. We're talking about three to six hours a week – or a minimum of thirty minutes a day, every other day. That hardly seems an inordinate amount of time considering the tremendous benefits in terms of the impact on the other 162 – 165 hours of the week. –Stephen Covey

147. When I lost all of my excuses, I found my results. –Unknown

148. Strength does not come from physical capacity. It comes from an indomitable will. —Mahatma Gandhi

149. The unfortunate thing about this world is that good habits are so much easier to give up than bad ones. —Somerset Maugham

150. Don't eat anything your great-great grandmother wouldn't recognize as food. There are a great many food-like items in the supermarket your ancestors wouldn't recognize as food... stay away from these. —Michael Pollan

151. I've missed more than 9,000 shots in my career. I've lost almost 300 games. Twenty-six times, I've been trusted to take the game winning shot and missed. I've failed over and over and over again in my life. And that is why I succeed. —Michael Jordan

152. If you want something you have never had, you have to do something you have never done. —Unknown

153. Bad habits are like a comfortable bed, easy to get into, but hard to get out of. —Unknown

154. Keep away from those who try to belittle your ambitions. Small people will always do that, but the really great people make you believe that you too can become great!
—Unknown

155. The first step toward success is taken when you refuse to be a captive of the environment in which you find yourself.
—Mark Caine

156. If I quit now, I will soon be back to where I started. When I started, I was desperate to get to where I am now. —Unknown

157. Hating your body will never get you as far as loving it will. —Unknown

158. Success is dependent upon the glands... the sweat glands. —Zig Ziglar

159. Every day, in every way, I am getting better and better. —Emilie Coue

160. You will never always be motivated. You have to learn to be disciplined. —Someone Smart

161. Your body can withstand almost anything. It's your mind that you have to convince! —Unknown

162. Whatever course you decide upon, there is always someone to tell you that you are wrong. There are always difficulties arising which tempt you to believe that your critics are right. To map out a course of action and follow it to an end requires courage. —Ralph Waldo Emerson

163. When I finish a workout, I feel pretty sexy. Even though I'm sweaty and I don't smell like a rose, I feel strong. It does a lot for me mentally and physically. —Sarah Shahi

164. A man's health can be judged by which he takes two at a time — pills or stairs. —Joan Welsh

165. There is nothing noble in being superior to someone else. The true nobility is in being superior to your previous self.
—Hindu Proverb

166. Don't stop when you're tired... stop when you are done! —Unknown

167. Want to learn to eat a lot? Here it is: Eat a little. That way, you will be around long enough to eat a lot.
—Anthony Robbins

168. The first thing you lose on a diet is your sense of humor. —Unknown

169. A man is born gentle and weak. At death, he is hard and stiff. Green plants are tender and filled with sap. At death, they are withered and dry. Therefore, the stiff and unbending is the disciple of death, and the gentle and yielding is the disciple of life. —Lao Tzu

170. Stop being afraid of what could go wrong, and start being excited about what could go right.
—Tony Robbins

171. You are intense. You are obsessed. You are not normal. You say *yes* when others say *no*. You rise while others sleep. You are better today than you were yesterday. You do what others will not do. You are in control of your destiny. —Unknown

172. Excuses are for people who don't want it enough. How bad do you want it? —K.J. Brady

173. Health is the greatest of all possessions; a pale cobbler is better than a sick king. —Isaac Bickerstaff

174. The harder you work for something, the greater you'll feel when you achieve it. —Unknown

175. You do not have to wait til January 1st to get healthy. You don't even have to wait til Monday. Start today. You will thank yourself 60 days from now. —Unknown

176. Don't you dare complain about your weight if you are doing nothing about it. —Your conscious

177. It never gets easier... you just get stronger. —Unknown

178. Think of your morning workouts as important meetings you have scheduled with yourself. Bosses don't cancel.
    —The Boss

179. I do not think that there is any other quality so essential to success of any kind as the quality of perseverance. It overcomes almost everything, even nature.
    —John D. Rockefeller

180. The same voice that says *"give up"* can also be trained to say *"keep going"*. —Unknown

181. I was never a natural athlete, but I paid my dues in sweat and concentration, and took the time necessary to learn karate and became a world champion. —Chuck Norris

182. The word aerobics comes from two Greek words: *aero*, meaning "ability to" and *bics*, meaning "withstand tremendous boredom". —Dave Barry

183. When you have a clear vision of your goal, it's easier to take the first step toward it. —L.L. Cool J

184. The secret of getting ahead
is getting started.
—Agatha Christie

185. Motivation will almost
always beat mere talent.
—Norman R. Augustine

186. I didn't count my sit-ups. I
only started counting
when it started to hurt
because those are the only
ones that count.
—Muhammad Ali

187. Courage doesn't always
roar. Sometimes courage is
the quiet voice at the end
of the day saying, "I will
try again tomorrow".
—Mary Anne Radmacher

188. With drive and a bit of talent, you can move mountains.
—Dwayne Johnson

189. Nothing can stop the man with the right mental attitude from achieving his goal; nothing on earth can help the man with the wrong mental attitude.
—Thomas Jefferson

190. Don't try to overhaul your life overnight. Instead, focus on making one small change at a time. Over time, those small changes will add up to a big transformation. Don't give up! —Unknown

191. Consistency: It's not about getting in beach body shape, but always "Beach Body ready".
   —Kizzito Ejam

192. Take care of your body. It's the only place you have to live. —Jim Rohn

193. Once you see results, it becomes an addiction.
   —Unknown

194. Push harder than yesterday if you want a different tomorrow.
   —Unknown

195. Life is tough, my darling, but so are you.
   -Stephanie Bennett-Henry

196. I know that if I set my mind to something, even if people are saying I can't do it, I will achieve it.
—David Beckham

197. What would you attempt to do if you knew you couldn't fail? —Unknown

198. Running is nothing more than a series of arguments between the part of your brain that wants to stop and the part that wants to keep going.
—Every Runner

199. The finish line is just the beginning of a whole new race. —Unknown

200. If you're fifty, exercise your mind and body regularly, eat well, and have a general zest for life, you're likely younger — in very real, physical terms — than your neighbor who is forty-four, works in a dead-end job, eats chicken wings twice a day, considers thinking too strenuous, and looks at lifting a beer glass as a reasonable daily workout.
   –Ken Robinson

201. I have not failed. I've just found 10,000 ways that won't work.
   –Thomas Edison

202. The last three or four reps is what makes the muscle grow. This area of pain divides the champion from someone else who is not a champion.
   —Arnold Schwarzenegger

203. Everyone faces defeat. It may be a stepping-stone or a stumbling block, depending on the mental attitude with which it is faced. —Napoleon Hill

204. Every day is another chance to get stronger, to eat better, to live healthier, and do the best version of you. —Unknown

205. Nothing worthwhile comes easily. Work, continuous work and hard work, is the only way to accomplish results that last.
—Hamilton Holt

206. What's my goal weight? I don't have one. I will not define myself by a number. My journey is about feeling strong, confident, and healthy. —Unknown

207. When it comes to eating right and exercising, there is no *"I'll start tomorrow"*. Tomorrow is disease.
—V.L. Allinear

208. Don't stop trying just because you hit a wall. Progress is still progress no matter how small.
—Unknown

209. It's not that some people have willpower and some don't. It's that some people are ready to change and others are not.
—James Gordon

210. Most diseases are the result of medication which has been prescribed to relieve and take away a beneficial and warning symptom on the part of nature.
—Elbert Hubbard

211. Every morning you have two choices: continue to sleep with your dreams, or to wake up and chase them. —Unknown

212. Your mind is a powerful thing. When you fill it with positive thoughts, your life will start to change. —Unknown

213. The best view comes after the hardest climb. —Unknown

214. Never let yourself get too comfortable. Seek challenges, push yourself, and ignore what others think. —Unknown

215. She was tempted to take the elevator instead of the stairs just this once. But that was how it started. Take the elevator tonight because she was tired and her feet hurt from having been trapped in three-inch stilettos all day, and then tomorrow she'd want to take it because she was running late. Then, the next thing she knew she'd be taking elevators all over the place because she got winded climbing stairs. —Melissa Miller

216. It always seems impossible until it's done. —Unknown

217. There is no traffic jam
along the extra mile.
—Roger Staubach

218. People with clear, written
goals accomplish far more
in a shorter period of time
than people without them
could ever imagine.
—Brian Tracy

219. If we could give every
individual the right
amount of nourishment
and exercise, not too little
and not too much, we
would have found the
safest way to health.
—Hippocrates

220. Ability is what you're capable of doing. Motivation determines what you do. Attitude determines how well you do it. —Lou Holtz

221. True healthcare reform starts in your kitchen, not in Washington. —Unknown

222. Never let your head hang down. Never give up and sit down and grieve. Find another way. —Satchel Paige

223. The best and most efficient pharmacy is within our own system. —Robert Peale

224. I've come to believe that all my past failure and frustration were actually laying the foundation for the understandings that have created the new level of living I now enjoy.
   —Anthony Robbins

225. There are seven days in the week and *someday* isn't one of them.
   —Unknown

226. We do not stop exercising because we grow old — we grow old because we stop exercising.
   —Dr. Kenneth Cooper

227. Health is like money, we never have a true idea of its value until we lose it. —Josh Billings

228. The next few months will go by no matter if you workout or not. Make them count! —Unknown

229. You dream. You plan. You reach. There will be obstacles. There will be doubters. There will be mistakes. But with hard work, with belief, with confidence and trust in yourself and those around you, there are no limits. —Michael Phelps

230. I'm not overweight. I'm just nine inches too short. —Shelley Winters

231. It is time to value physical education as a core subject in schools, as it plays a critical role in teaching students how to achieve optimal health and physical fitness, while increasing their ability to succeed academically. —Elissa Bassler

232. Sweat is just your fat crying. —Unknown

233. The difference between a goal and a dream is a deadline. —Steve Smith

234. Life has its ups and downs... we call them squats. —Unknown

235. It's never too late to become what you might have been. —George Eliot

236. There is no one giant step that does it, it's a lot of little steps. —Peter Cohen

237. Life expectancy would grow by leaps and bounds if green vegetables smelled as good as bacon. —Doug Larson

238. If you need motivation to lose weight, just go eat in front of the mirror while you are naked. —Unknown

239. The ingredients of health and long life are: great temperance, open air, easy labor, and little care. —Sir Phillip Sidney

240. He who enjoys good health is rich, though he knows it not. —Italian Proverb

241. Yes, you should try to eat healthy. No, you should not be on a diet. You should eat healthy all the time. —Unknown

242. There is no shortcut. It takes time to build a better, stronger version of yourself. —Unknown

243. Don't try to be perfect.
Just try and be better
than you were yesterday.
—Unknown

244. Fear is what stops you...
courage is what keeps you
going. —Unknown

245. There will be haters, there
will be doubters, there will
be non-believers, and then
there will be you... proving
them all wrong.
—Unknown

246. To keep the body in good
health is a duty...
otherwise we shall not be
able to keep our mind
strong and clear. —Buddha

247. Today is my tomorrow. It's up to me to shape it, to take control and to seize every opportunity. The power is in the choices I make each and every day. I eat well, I live well. I shape me! —Unknown

248. The body achieves what the mind believes. —Napoleon Hill

249. The next few months could be a period of magnificent transformation... make the most of them. —Unknown

250. Unless you puke, faint or die, keep going! —Jillian Michaels

251. The man who removes a mountain begins by carrying away small stones. —William Faulkner

252. My temptation is emotional, and resisting will further my needed weight loss and strengthen my character. Furthermore, nothing tastes as good as thin feels. —Stephen Covey

253. I have two doctors, my left leg and my right. —G.M. Trevelyan

254. Tomorrow is often the busiest day of the week. —Spanish Proverb

255. The one who falls and gets up is so much stronger than the one who never fell. —Unknown

256. There comes a certain point in life when you have to stop blaming other people for how you feel or the misfortunes in your life. You can't go through life obsessing about what might have been. —Hugh Jackman

257. You can, you should, and if you're brave enough to start, you will. —Stephen King

258. Fitness is not about being better than someone else, it's about being better than you used to be. —Unknown

259. You must expect great things of yourself before you can do them. —Michael Jordan

260. You have to put in many, many, many tiny efforts that nobody sees or appreciates before you achieve anything worthwhile. —Brian Tracy

261. No matter how slow you go, you are still lapping everyone on the couch! —Unknown

262. Train like an athlete, eat like a nutritionist, sleep like a baby, win like a champion. —Unknown

263. "I don't have time" is the adult version of "The dog ate my homework". —Unknown

264. You'll get a lot more compliments for working out than you will for sleeping in. —Unknown

265. The only way to keep your health is to eat what you don't want, drink what you don't like, and do what you'd rather not. —Mark Twain

266. If you find a path with no obstacles, it probably doesn't lead anywhere. —Unknown

267. Physical fitness is not only one of the most important keys to a healthy body, it's the basis of a dynamic and creative intellectual activity. —John F. Kennedy

268. Be thankful for what you are now, and keep fighting for what you want to be tomorrow. —Unknown

269. Our bodies are our gardens, and our wills are our gardeners. —William Shakespeare

270. He who takes medicine and neglects to watch his diet wastes the skill of his doctors. —Chinese proverb

271. I know the price of success: dedication, hard work and an unremitting devotion to the things you want to see happen.
—Frank Lloyd Wright

272. Health is a state of complete harmony of the body, mind, and spirit. When one is free from physical disabilities and mental distractions, the gates of the soul open.
—B.K.S. Iyengar

273. What consumes your mind will ultimately control your life. —Unknown

274. Why would you choose to fail when success is an option? —Jillian Michaels

275. The reason most people never reach their goals is that they don't define them, or ever seriously consider them as believable or achievable. Winners can tell you where they are going, what they plan to do along the way, and who will be sharing the adventure with them. —Denis Waitley

276. If it weren't for the fact that the TV set and the refrigerator are so far apart, some of us wouldn't get any exercise at all.
    —Joey Adams

277. Excuses don't burn calories.
    —Unknown

278. Strong people are harder to kill than weak people and are more useful in general. —Mark Rippetoe

279. There's lots of people in this world who spend so much time watching their health that they haven't the time to enjoy it.
    —Josh Billings

280. If it was easy, everyone would do it. —Unknown

281. Anyone can work out for an hour, but to control what goes on your plate the other 23 hours... that's the hard work! —Unknown

282. Try a thing you haven't done three times. Once to get over the fear of doing it. Twice to learn how to do it. And a third time to figure out whether you like it or not. —Joyce Meyer

283. Energy and persistence conquer all things.
     —Benjamin Franklin

284. You're going to have to let it hurt. Let it suck. The harder you work, the better you will look. Your appearance isn't parallel to how heavy you lift, it's parallel to how hard you work. —Joe Manganiello

285. Never mistake activity for achievement.
—John Wooden

286. Some things you have to do every day. Eating seven apples on Saturday night instead of one a day just isn't going to get the job done. —Jim Rohn

287. Those who think they have no time for bodily exercise will sooner or later have to find time for illness.
—Edward Stanley

288. When I'm running I don't have to talk to anyone and don't have to listen to anyone. This is a part of my day I can't do without.
—Haruki Marukami

289. Nothing great was ever achieved without enthusiasm.
—Ralph Waldo Emerson

290. You are always only one workout away from a good mood. —Unknown

291. The higher your energy level, the more efficient your body. The more efficient your body, the better you feel and the more you will use your talent to produce outstanding results.
—Anthony Robbins

292. Move out of your comfort zone. You can only grow if you are willing to feel awkward and uncomfortable when you try something new.
—Brian Tracy

293. If you can't pronounce it, don't eat it!
—Common Sense

294. If it doesn't challenge you, it doesn't change you. —Fred Devito

295. Don't give up because of what someone said. Use that as motivation to push you harder! —Unknown

296. How do you want to feel when summer rolls around... fit or jealous? —Unknown

297. A goal without a plan is just a wish. —Larry Elde

298. Winners are not people who never fail, but people who never quit. Be a winner. —Unknown

299. The doctor of the future will no longer treat the human frame with drugs, but rather will cure and prevent disease with nutrition. —Thomas Edison

300. Fitness is 20% exercise and 80% nutrition. You can't outrun your fork.
—Unknown

301. You must take personal responsibility. You cannot change the circumstances, the seasons, or the wind, but you can change yourself. —Jim Rohn

302. I regret that *working*.
—No one, ever

303. Be miserable. Or motivate yourself. Whatever has to be done, it's always your choice. —Wayne Dyer

304. He who cures a disease may be the skillfullest, but he that prevents it is the safest physician.
—Thomas Fuller

305. If you are going through hell keep going.
—Winston Churchill

306. Don't dig your grave with your own knife and fork.
—English Proverb

307. It's a slow process, don't make it slower by quitting.
—Unknown

308. I never dreamt of success. I worked for it.
   —Estee Lauder

309. Motivation is a fire from within. If someone else tries to light that fire under you, chances are it will burn very briefly.
   —Stephen R. Covey

310. It takes 21 days. 21 days of healthy eating and working out and it will become a habit. —Unknown

311. If you aren't hungry enough to eat an apple, you're not really hungry, you are just bored.
   —Unknown

312. If you are tired of starting over, stop giving up.
    —Unknown

313. It's better to take many small steps in the right direction than to make a great leap forward only to stumble backward.
    —Chinese proverb

314. Few people know how to take a walk. The qualifications are endurance, plain clothes, old shoes, an eye for nature, good humor, vast curiosity, good speech, good silence and nothing too much.
    —Ralph Waldo Emerson

315. Age is no barrier. It's a limitation you put on your mind.
    —Jackie Joyner-Kersee

316. Learn to relax. Your body is precious, as it houses your mind and spirit. Inner peace begins with a relaxed body.
    —Norman Vincent Peale

317. It is never too late to get your shit together!
    —Unknown

318. From the bitterness of disease, man learns the sweetness of health.
    —Catalan proverb

319. You want me to do something.... tell me I can't do it. —Maya Angelou

320. Fall in love with the process and the results will come. —Unknown

321. You will never know your limits unless you push yourself to them. —Unknown

322. I want to inspire people. I want someone to look at me and say *"because of you, I didn't quit"*. —Unknown

323. Your body is a temple, but only if you treat it as one. —Astrid Alauda

324. You have to push past your perceived limits, push past that point you thought was as far as you can go. —Drew Brees

325. The real workout starts when you want to stop! —Unknown

326. Living a healthy lifestyle will only deprive you of poor health, lethargy, and fat. —Jill Johnson

327. Sometimes the smallest step in the right direction ends up being the biggest step of your life. —Unknown

328. The more you eat, the less flavor. The less you eat, the more flavor.
—Chinese Proverb

329. A lot of times people look at the negative side of what they feel they can't do. I always look on the positive side of what I can do. —Chuck Norris

330. A good laugh and a long sleep are the best cures in the doctor's book.
—Irish Proverb

331. You miss 100% of the shots you don't take.
—Wayne Gretsky

332. Do yourself a favor, and realize that there's no technique in the world that will save you. There are no pills, no secrets, no passwords on the path to greatness. You've got to embrace the pain, push the threshold, and feel the suck, and then you've got to muster the courage to go back six times a week. —Jon Gilson

333. Don't put a deadline on your body. You have your entire life to be healthy and happy. Losing 20 pounds in 30 days doesn't mean anything. —Unknown

334. You can feel sore tomorrow or you can feel sorry tomorrow. You choose. —Unknown

335. Eat clean, stay fit, and have a burger to stay sane. —Gigi Hadid

336. No discipline is enjoyable while it is happening, it's painful! But afterwards there will be a peaceful harvest of right living for those who are trained in this way. —Hebrews 12:11

337. The road to success is dotted with many tempting parking places. —Unknown

338. The truth is that our finest moments are most likely to occur when we are feeling deeply uncomfortable, unhappy, or unfulfilled. For it is only in such moments, propelled by our discomfort, that we are likely to step out of our ruts and start searching for different ways or truer answers. —M. Scott

339. You've always been beautiful. Now you're just deciding to be healthier, fitter, faster, and stronger. Remember that.
—Unknown

340. Instead of saying "I don't have time" try saying "It's not a priority" and see how that feels. —Unknown

341. The fact that you aren't where you want to be should be motivation enough. —Unknown

342. Don't diet. Just eat according to your goals. —Unknown

343. The difference between someone who is in shape and someone who is not in shape is the individual who is in shape works out even when they do not want to. —Unknown

344. Health is the first muse
and sleep is the condition
to produce it.
    −Ralph Waldo Emerson

345. Early to bed and early to
rise, makes a man healthy,
wealthy and wise.
    −Benjamin Franklin

346. Stand up to your obstacles
and do something about
them. You will find that
they haven't half the
strength you think they
have.
    −Norman Vincent Peale

347. The physically fit can enjoy
their vices. −Lord Percival

348. You may only succeed if you desire succeeding; you may only fail if you do not mind failing. —Philippos

349. Don't think about what can happen in a month. Don't think about what can happen in a year. Just focus on the 24 hours in front of you and do what you can do to get closer to where you want to be. —Unknown

350. Real difficulties can be overcome; it is only the imaginary ones that are unconquerable. —Theodore N. Vail

351. What is the point of being alive if you don't at least try to do something remarkable? —Unknown

352. Who cares if you have said you were going to get in shape 100 times and quit 100 times. Say it again, and this time don't quit. Your past doesn't decide your future... you do. —Unknown

353. It's bizarre that the produce manager is more important to my children's health than the pediatrician. —Meryl Streep

354. Our food should be our medicine and our medicine should be our food.
—Hippocrates

355. I hated every minute of training, but I said *"don't quit"*! Suffer now and live the rest of your life as a champion.
—Muhammad Ali

356. If you are surprised at the number of maladies, count our cooks. —Seneca

357. Food is the most abused anxiety drug. Exercise is the most underutilized antidepressant.
—Bill Phillips

358. Remember how: your clothes don't fit, your body feels sluggish, your skin doesn't glow, you don't have the energy, you want to feel beautiful, you're regretting what you ate, you wished you had worked out, you wanted to change... before making another unhealthy choice. —Unknown

359. If you get tired, learn to rest, not quit. —Unknown

360. One of the greatest moments in life is realizing that two weeks ago your body couldn't do what it just did. —Unknown

361. So many people spend their health gaining wealth, and then have to spend their wealth to regain their health. —A.J. Materi

362. Suck it up. And one day you won't have to suck it in. —Unknown

363. It's not whether you get knocked down, it's whether you get up. —Vince Lombardi

364. You believe in yourself when no one else does. That makes you a winner right there. —Venus Williams

365. Success isn't given, it's earned. On the track, on the field, in the weight room. With blood, sweat, and the occasional tear. —Unknown

366. Yoga teaches us to cure what need not be endured and endure what cannot be cured. —B.K.S. Iyengar

367. Once you can control your mind, you can conquer your body. —Unknown

368. I don't have time for hobbies. At the end of the day, I treat my job as a hobby. It's something I love doing. —David Beckham

369. You measure the size of the accomplishment by the obstacles you had to overcome to reach your goals.
—Booker T. Washington

370. I once cried because I had no shoes to play soccer, but one day, I met a man who had no feet.
—Zinedine Zidane

371. The secret is to believe in your dreams, in your potential that you can be like your star, keep searching, keep believing and don't lose faith in yourself. -Neymar

372. What to do with a mistake: recognize it, admit it, learn from it, forget it. —Dean Smith

373. You find that you have peace of mind and can enjoy yourself, get more sleep, and rest when you know that it was a one hundred percent effort that you gave — win or lose. —Gordie Howe

374. You can motivate by fear, and you can motivate by reward. But both of those methods are only temporary. The only lasting thing is self-motivation. —Homer Rice

375. What you lack in talent can be made up with desire, hustle, and giving 110 percent all the time.
    —Don Zimmer

376. Continuous effort — not strength or intelligence — is the key to unlocking your potential.
    —Liane Cardes

377. In baseball and in business, there are three types of people. Those who make it happen, those who watch it happen, and those who wonder what happened.
    —Tommy Lasorda

378. The more difficult the victory, the greater the happiness in winning.
—Pele

379. Eat better. Run more. Squat more. Sleep earlier. Wake up earlier. Make a good breakfast. Drink a lot of water. Eat fruits. Read books. Adventure. Talk less. Listen more. Feel deeper. Love better. Open your eyes. Experience Life. Be happy. —Someone Smart

Well, you have reached the end of this book. It has been very difficult trying to narrow it down to my favorite quotes of all time. I hope that these quotes helped you on days where you needed an extra boost to maximize your success.

P.S. I added in a couple of bonus quotes for you, mostly because I couldn't get all the way down to the final 365. I hope you enjoyed them! :)

This book is also available for digital download if you would like to keep it on your phone or tablet for quick reference or for a little pocket motivation.

Please visit us at www.littlebookofquotes.com